The Ultimate Keto Vegan Delicacies Book

Boost your metabolism and your brain with these irresistible keto vegan recipes

Susan Muncy

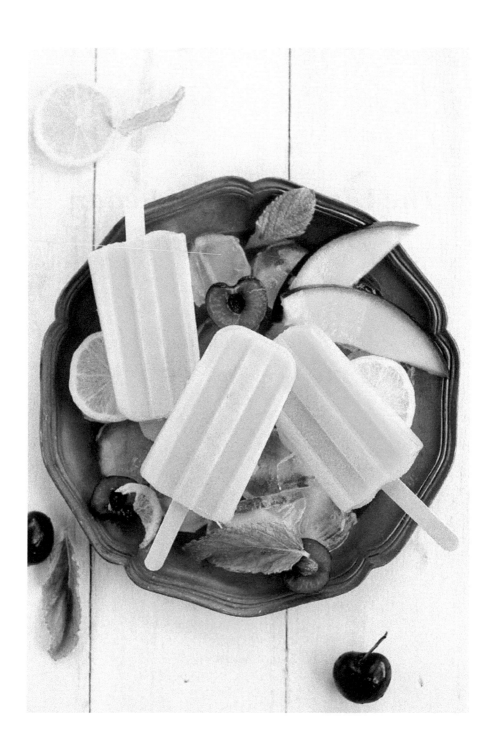

3

Table of Contents

Ginger Smoothie with Citrus and Mint

Preparation Time: 5 minutes

Cooking Time: 3 minutes

Servings: 3

Ingredients:

- 1 head Romaine lettuce, chopped into 4 chunks
- 2 Tbsp. hemp seeds
- 5 mandarin oranges, peeled
- 1 banana, frozen
- 1 carrot
- 2-3 mint leaves
- ½ piece ginger root, peeled
- 1 cup water
- ¼ lemon, peeled
- ½ cup ice

Directions:

1. Put all the smoothie ingredients in a blender and blend until smooth.
2. Enjoy!

Nutrition: Calories 101 Fat 4 g Carbohydrates 14 g Sugar 1 g Protein 2 g Cholesterol 3 mg

Strawberry Beet Smoothie

Preparation Time: 5 minutes

Cooking Time: 50 minutes

Servings: 2

Ingredients:

- 1 red beet, trimmed, peeled and chopped into cubes
- 1 cup strawberries, quartered
- 1 ripe banana
- ½ cup strawberry yoghurt
- 1 Tbsp. honey
- 1 Tbsp. water
- Milk, to taste

Directions:

1. Sprinkle the beet cubes with water, place on aluminum foil and put in the oven (preheated to 204°C). Bake for 40 minutes.
2. Let the baked beet cool.
3. Combine all the smoothie ingredients.
4. Enjoy your fantastic drink.

Nutrition: Calories 184 Fat 9.2 g Carbohydrates 1 g Sugar 0.4 g Protein 24.9 g Cholesterol 132 mg

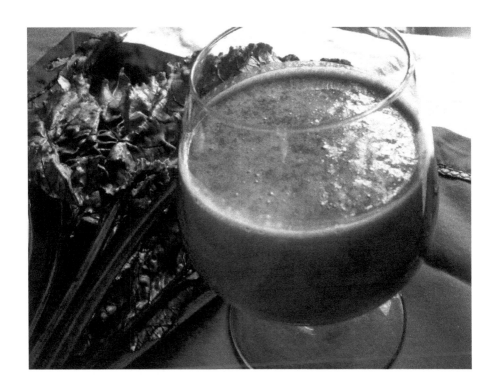

Peanut Butter Shake

Preparation Time: 5 minutes

Cooking Time: 5 minutes

Servings: 2

Ingredients:

- 1 cup plant-based milk
- 1 handful kale
- 2 bananas, frozen
- 2 Tbsp. peanut butter
- ½ tsp ground cinnamon
- ¼ tsp vanilla powder

Directions:

1. Use a blender to combine all the ingredients for your shake.
2. Enjoy it!

Nutrition: Calories 184 Fat 9.2 g Carbohydrates 1 g Sugar 0.4 g Protein 24.9 g Cholesterol 132 mg

Chocolate and Avocado Pudding

Preparation Time: 3 hours and 10 minutes

Cooking Time: 0 minute

Servings: 1

Ingredients:

- 1 small avocado, pitted, peeled
- 1 small banana, mashed
- 1/3 cup cocoa powder, unsweetened
- 1 tablespoon cacao nibs, unsweetened
- 1/4 cup maple syrup
- 1/3 cup coconut cream

Directions:

1. Add avocado in a food processor along with cream and then pulse for 2 minutes until smooth.
2. Add remaining ingredients, blend until mixed, and then tip the pudding in a container.
3. Cover the container with a plastic wrap; it should touch the pudding and refrigerate for 3 hours.
4. Serve straight away.

Nutrition: Calories: 87 Cal Fat: 7 g Carbs: 9 g Protein: 1.5 g Fiber: 3.2 g

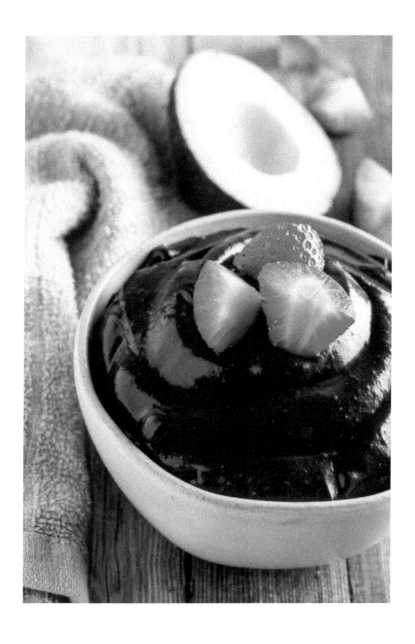

Chocolate Avocado Ice Cream

Preparation Time: 1 hour and 10 minutes

Cooking Time: 0 minute

Servings: 2

Ingredients:

- 4.5 ounces avocado, peeled, pitted
- 1/2 cup cocoa powder, unsweetened
- 1 tablespoon vanilla extract, unsweetened
- 1/2 cup and 2 tablespoons maple syrup
- 13.5 ounces coconut milk, unsweetened
- 1/2 cup water

Directions:

1. Add avocado in a food processor along with milk and then pulse for 2 minutes until smooth.
2. Add remaining ingredients, blend until mixed, and then tip the pudding in a freezer-proof container.
3. Place the container in a freezer and chill for freeze for 4 hours until firm, whisking every 20 minutes after 1 hour.

4. Serve straight away.

Nutrition: Calories: 80.7 Cal Fat: 7.1 g Carbs: 6 g Protein: 0.6 g Fiber: 2 g

Watermelon Mint Popsicles

Preparation Time: 8 hours and 5 minutes

Cooking Time: 0 minute

Servings: 8

Ingredients:

- 20 mint leaves, diced
- 6 cups watermelon chunks
- 3 tablespoons lime juice

Directions:

1. Add watermelon in a food processor along with lime juice and then pulse for 15 seconds until smooth.

2. Pass the watermelon mixture through a strainer placed over a bowl, remove the seeds and then stir mint into the collected watermelon mixture.

3. Take eight Popsicle molds, pour in prepared watermelon mixture, and freeze for 2 hours until slightly firm.

4. Then insert popsicle sticks and continue freezing for 6 hours until solid.

5. Serve straight away

Nutrition: Calories: 90 Cal Fat: 0 g Carbs: 23 g Protein: 0 g Fiber: 0 g

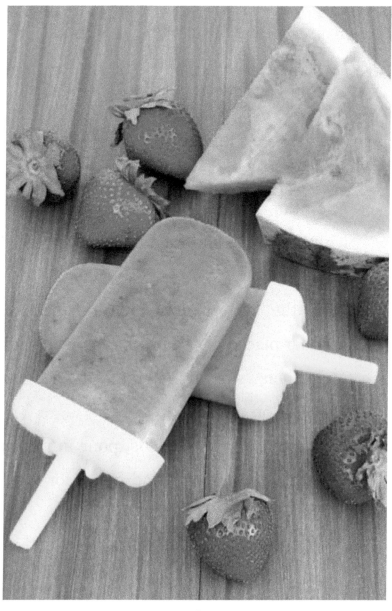

Brownie Energy Bites

Preparation Time: 1 hour and 10 minutes

Cooking Time: 0 minute

Servings: 2

Ingredients:

- 1/2 cup walnuts
- 1 cup Medjool dates, chopped
- 1/2 cup almonds
- 1/8 teaspoon salt
- 1/2 cup shredded coconut flakes
- 1/3 cup and 2 teaspoons cocoa powder, unsweetened

Directions:

1. Place almonds and walnuts in a food processor and pulse for 3 minutes until the dough starts to come together.
2. Add remaining ingredients, reserving ¼ cup of coconut and pulse for 2 minutes until incorporated.

3. Shape the mixture into balls, roll them in remaining coconut until coated, and refrigerate for 1 hour.

4. Serve straight away

Nutrition: Calories: 174.6 Cal Fat: 8.1 g Carbs: 25.5 g Protein: 4.1 g Fiber: 4.4 g

Salted Caramel Chocolate Cups

Preparation Time: 5 minutes

Cooking Time: 2 minutes

Servings: 12

Ingredients:

- ¼ teaspoon sea salt granules
- 1 cup dark chocolate chips, unsweetened
- 2 teaspoons coconut oil
- 6 tablespoons caramel sauce

Directions:

1. Take a heatproof bowl, add chocolate chips and oil, stir until mixed, then microwave for 1 minute until melted, stir chocolate and continue heating in the microwave for 30 seconds.

2. Take twelve mini muffin tins, line them with muffin liners, spoon a little bit of chocolate mixture into the tins, spread the chocolate in the bottom and along the sides, and freeze for 10 minutes until set.

3. Then fill each cup with ½ tablespoon of caramel sauce, cover with remaining chocolate and freeze for another 2salto minutes until set.

4. When ready to eat, peel off liner from the cup, sprinkle with sauce, and serve.

Nutrition: Calories: 80 Cal Fat: 5 g Carbs: 10 g Protein: 1 g Fiber: 0.5 g

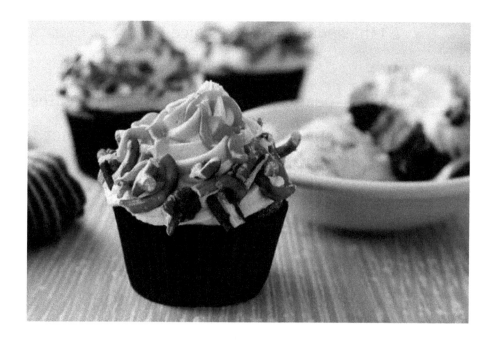

Chocolate Peanut Butter Energy Bites

Preparation Time: 1 hour and 5 minutes

Cooking Time: 0 minute

Servings: 4

Ingredients:

- 1/2 cup oats, old-fashioned
- 1/3 cup cocoa powder, unsweetened
- 1 cup dates, chopped
- 1/2 cup shredded coconut flakes, unsweetened
- 1/2 cup peanut butter

Directions:

1. Place oats in a food processor along with dates and pulse for 1 minute until the paste starts to come together.
2. Then add remaining ingredients, and blend until incorporated and very thick mixture comes together.
3. Shape the mixture into balls, refrigerate for 1 hour until set and then serve.

Nutrition: Calories: 88.6 Cal Fat: 5 g Carbs: 10 g Protein: 2.3 g Fiber: 1.6 g

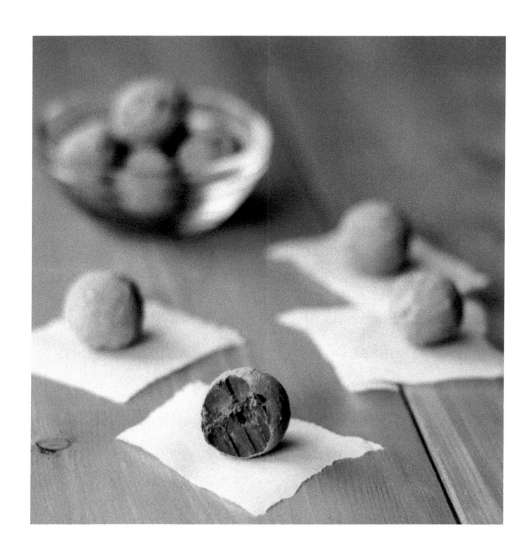

Cookie Dough Bites

Preparation Time: 4 hours and 10 minutes

Cooking Time: 0 minute

Servings: 18

Ingredients:

- 15 ounces cooked chickpeas
- 1/3 cup vegan chocolate chips
- 1/3 cup and 2 tablespoons peanut butter
- 8 Medjool dates pitted
- 1 teaspoon vanilla extract, unsweetened
- 2 tablespoons maple syrup
- 1 1/2 tablespoons almond milk, unsweetened

Directions:

1. Place chickpeas in a food processor along with dates, butter, and vanilla and then process for 2 minutes until smooth.

2. Add remaining ingredients, except for chocolate chips, and then pulse for 1 minute until blends and dough comes together.

3. Add chocolate chips, stir until just mixed, and then shape the mixture into 18 balls and refrigerate for 4 hours until firm.

4. Serve straight away

Nutrition: Calories: 200 Cal Fat: 9 g Carbs: 26 g Protein: 1 g Fiber: 0 g

Dark Chocolate Bars

Preparation Time: 1 hour and 10 minutes

Cooking Time: 2 minutes

Servings: 12

Ingredients:

- 1 cup cocoa powder, unsweetened
- 3 Tablespoons cacao nibs
- 1/8 teaspoon sea salt
- 2 Tablespoons maple syrup
- 1 1/4 cup chopped cocoa butter
- 1/2 teaspoons vanilla extract, unsweetened
- 2 Tablespoons coconut oil

Directions:

1. Take a heatproof bowl, add butter, oil, stir, and microwave for 90 to 120 seconds until melts, stirring every 30 seconds.

2. Sift cocoa powder over melted butter mixture, whisk well until combined, and then stir in maple syrup, vanilla, and salt until mixed.

3. Distribute the mixture evenly between twelve mini cupcake liners, top with cacao nibs, and freeze for 1 hour until set.

4. Serve straight away

Nutrition: Calories: 100 Cal Fat: 9 g Carbs: 8 g Protein: 2 g Fiber: 2 g

Almond Butter, Oat and Protein Energy Balls

Preparation Time: 1 hour and 10 minutes

Cooking Time: 3 minutes

Servings: 4

Ingredients:

- 1 cup rolled oats
- ½ cup honey
- 2 ½ scoops of vanilla protein powder
- 1 cup almond butter
- Chia seeds for rolling

Directions:

1. Take a skillet pan, place it over medium heat, add butter and honey, stir and cook for 2 minutes until warm.

2. Transfer the mixture into a bowl, stir in protein powder until mixed, and then stir in oatmeal until combined.

3. Shape the mixture into balls, roll them into chia seeds, then arrange them on a cookie sheet and refrigerate for 1 hour until firm.

4. Serve straight away

Nutrition: Calories: 200 Cal Fat: 10 g Carbs: 21 g Protein: 7 g Fiber: 4 g

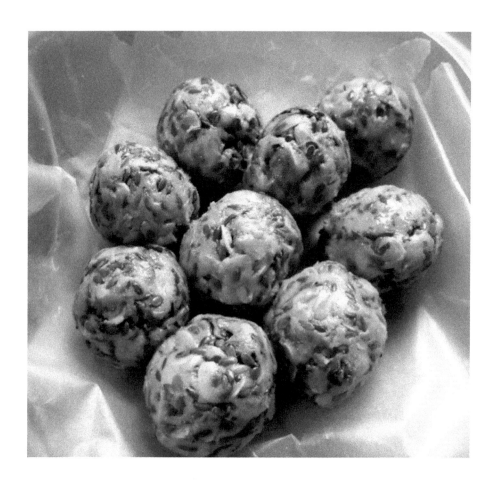

Chocolate and Avocado Truffles

Preparation Time: 1 hour and 10 minutes

Cooking Time: 1 minute

Servings: 18

Ingredients:

- 1 medium avocado, ripe
- 2 tablespoons cocoa powder
- 10 ounces of dark chocolate chips

Directions:

1. Scoop out the flesh from avocado, place it in a bowl, then mash with a fork until smooth, and stir in 1/2 cup chocolate chips.
2. Place remaining chocolate chips in a heatproof bowl and microwave for 1 minute until chocolate has melted, stirring halfway.
3. Add melted chocolate into avocado mixture, stir well until blended, and then refrigerate for 1 hour.
4. Then shape the mixture into balls, 1 tablespoon of mixture per ball, and roll in cocoa powder until covered.

5. Serve straight away.

Nutrition: Calories: 59 Cal Fat: 4 g Carbs: 7 g Protein: 0 g Fiber: 1 g

Coconut Oil Cookies

Preparation Time: 10 minutes

Cooking Time: 10 minutes

Servings: 15

Ingredients:

- 3 1/4 cup oats
- 1/2 teaspoons salt
- 2 cups coconut Sugar
- 1 teaspoons vanilla extract, unsweetened
- 1/4 cup cocoa powder
- 1/2 cup liquid Coconut Oil
- 1/2 cup peanut butter
- 1/2 cup cashew milk

Directions:

1. Take a saucepan, place it over medium heat, add all the ingredients except for oats and vanilla, stir until mixed, and then bring the mixture to boil.

2. Simmer the mixture for 4 minutes, mixing frequently, then remove the pan from heat and stir in vanilla.

3. Add oats, stir until well mixed and then scoop the mixture on a plate lined with wax paper.

4. Serve straight away.

Nutrition: Calories: 112 Cal Fat: 6.5 g Carbs: 13 g Protein: 1.4 g Fiber: 0.1 g

Apple Crumble

Preparation Time: 20 minutes

Cooking Time: 25 minutes

Servings: 6

Ingredients:

- For the filling
- 4 to 5 apples, cored and chopped (about 6 cups)
- ½ cup unsweetened applesauce, or ¼ cup water
- 2 to 3 tablespoons unrefined sugar (coconut, date, sucanat, maple syrup)
- 1 teaspoon ground cinnamon
- Pinch sea salt
- For the crumble
- 2 tablespoons almond butter, or cashew or sunflower seed butter
- 2 tablespoons maple syrup
- 1½ cups rolled oats
- ½ cup walnuts, finely chopped

- ½ teaspoon ground cinnamon
- 2 to 3 tablespoons unrefined granular sugar (coconut, date, sucanat)

Directions:

1. Preparing the Ingredients.
2. Preheat the oven to 350°F. Put the apples and applesauce in an 8-inch-square baking dish, and sprinkle with the sugar, cinnamon, and salt. Toss to combine.
3. In a medium bowl, mix together the nut butter and maple syrup until smooth and creamy. Add the oats, walnuts, cinnamon, and sugar and stir to coat, using your hands if necessary. (If you have a small food processor, pulse the oats and walnuts together before adding them to the mix.)
4. Sprinkle the topping over the apples and put the dish in the oven.
5. Bake for 20 to 25 minutes, or until the fruit is soft and the topping is lightly browned.

Nutrition: Calories 195 Fat 7 g Carbohydrates 6 g Sugar 2 g Protein 24 g Cholesterol 65 mg

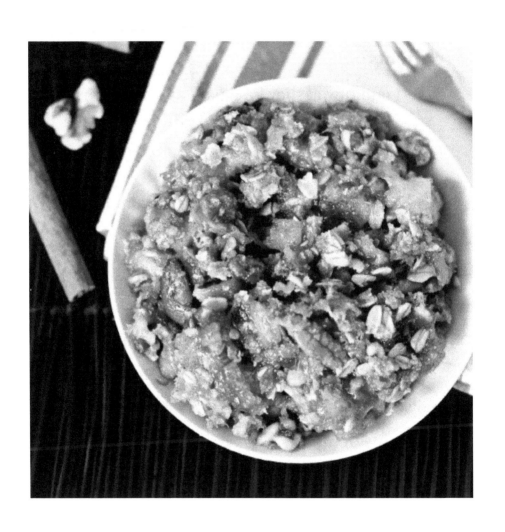

Cashew-Chocolate Truffles

Preparation Time: 15 minutes

Cooking Time: 0 minutes

Servings: 12

Ingredients:

- 1 cup raw cashews, soaked in water overnight
- ¾ cup pitted dates
- 2 tablespoons coconut oil
- 1 cup unsweetened shredded coconut, divided
- 1 to 2 tablespoons cocoa powder, to taste

Directions:

1. Preparing the Ingredients.
2. In a food processor, combine the cashews, dates, coconut oil, ½ cup of shredded coconut, and cocoa powder. Pulse until fully incorporated; it will resemble chunky cookie dough. Spread the remaining ½ cup of shredded coconut on a plate.
3. Form the mixture into tablespoon-size balls and roll on the plate to cover with the shredded coconut. Transfer to a parchment paper–lined plate or baking sheet. Repeat to make 12 truffles.

4. Place the truffles in the refrigerator for 1 hour to set. Transfer the truffles to a storage container or freezer-safe bag and seal.

Nutrition: Calories 160 Fat 1 g Carbohydrates 1 g Sugar 0.5 g Protein 22 g Cholesterol 60 mg

Banana Chocolate Cupcakes

Preparation Time: 20 minutes

Cooking Time: 20 minutes

Servings: 1

Ingredients:

- 3 medium bananas
- 1 cup non-dairy milk
- 2 tablespoons almond butter
- 1 teaspoon apple cider vinegar
- 1 teaspoon pure vanilla extract
- 1¼ cups whole-grain flour
- ½ cup rolled oats
- ¼ cup coconut sugar (optional)
- 1 teaspoon baking powder
- ½ teaspoon baking soda
- ½ cup unsweetened cocoa powder
- ¼ cup chia seeds, or sesame seeds
- Pinch sea salt
- ¼ cup dark chocolate chips, dried cranberries, or raisins (optional)

Directions:

1. Preparing the Ingredients.

2. Preheat the oven to 350°F. Lightly grease the cups of two 6-cup muffin tins or line with paper muffin cups.

3. Put the bananas, milk, almond butter, vinegar, and vanilla in a blender and purée until smooth. Or stir together in a large bowl until smooth and creamy.

4. Put the flour, oats, sugar (if using), baking powder, baking soda, cocoa powder, chia seeds, salt, and chocolate chips in another large bowl, and stir to combine. Mix together the wet and dry ingredients, stirring as little as possible. Spoon into muffin cups and bake for 20 to 25 minutes. Take the cupcakes out of the oven and let them cool fully before taking out of the muffin tins, since they will be very moist.

Nutrition: Calories 295 Fat 17 g Carbohydrates 4 g Sugar 0.1 g Protein 29 g Cholesterol 260 mg

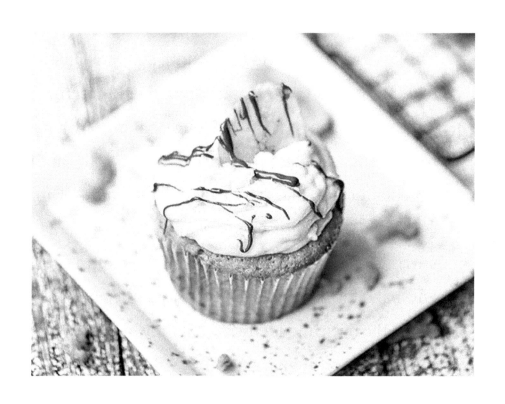

Minty Fruit Salad

Preparation Time: 15 minutes

Cooking Time: 5 minutes

Servings: 4

Ingredients:

- ¼ cup lemon juice (about 2 small lemons)
- 4 teaspoons maple syrup or agave syrup
- 2 cups chopped pineapple
- 2 cups chopped strawberries
- 2 cups raspberries
- 1 cup blueberries
- 8 fresh mint leaves

Directions:

Preparing the Ingredients.

1. Beginning with 1 mason jar, add the ingredients in this order:

2. 1 tablespoon of lemon juice, 1 teaspoon of maple syrup, ½ cup of pineapple, ½ cup of strawberries, ½ cup of raspberries, ¼ cup of blueberries, and 2 mint leaves.

3. Repeat to fill 3 more jars. Close the jars tightly with lids.

4. Place the airtight jars in the refrigerator for up to 3 days.

Nutrition: Calories 339 Fat 17.5 g Carbohydrates 2 g Sugar 2 g Protein 44 g Cholesterol 100 mg

Cherry-Vanilla Rice Pudding (Pressure cooker)

Preparation Time: 5 minutes

Cooking Time: 30 minutes

Servings: 4-6

Ingredients:

- 1 cup short-grain brown rice
- 1¾ cups nondairy milk, plus more as needed
- 1½ cups water
- 4 tablespoons unrefined sugar or pure maple syrup (use 2 tablespoons if you use a sweetened milk), plus more as needed
- 1 teaspoon vanilla extract (use ½ teaspoon if you use vanilla milk)
- Pinch salt
- ¼ cup dried cherries or ½ cup fresh or frozen pitted cherries

Directions:

1. Preparing the Ingredients. In your electric pressure cooker's cooking pot, combine the rice, milk, water, sugar, vanilla, and salt.

2. High pressure for 30 minutes. Close and lock the lid and select High Pressure for 30 minutes.

3. Pressure Release. Once the Cooking Time is complete, let the pressure release naturally, about 20 minutes. Unlock and remove the lid. Stir in the cherries and put the lid back on loosely for about 10 minutes. Serve, adding more milk or sugar, as desired.

Nutrition: Calories 420 Fat 27.4 g Carbohydrates 2 g Sugar 0.3 g Protein 46.3 g Cholesterol 98 mg

Peach-Mango Crumble (Pressure cooker)

Preparation Time: 10 minutes

Cooking Time: 6 minutes

Servings: 4-6

Ingredient:

- 3 cups chopped fresh or frozen peaches
- 3 cups chopped fresh or frozen mangos
- 4 tablespoons unrefined sugar or pure maple syrup, divided
- 1 cup gluten-free rolled oats
- ½ cup shredded coconut, sweetened or unsweetened
- 2 tablespoons coconut oil or vegan margarine

Directions:

1. Preparing the Ingredients. In a 6- to 7-inch round baking dish, toss together the peaches, mangos, and 2 tablespoons of sugar. In a food processor, combine the oats, coconut, coconut oil, and remaining 2 tablespoons of sugar. Pulse until combined. (If you use maple syrup, you'll need less coconut oil. Start with just the syrup and add oil if

the mixture is not sticking together.) Sprinkle the oat mixture over the fruit mixture.

2. Cover the dish with aluminum foil. Put a trivet in the bottom of your electric pressure cooker's cooking pot and pour in a cup or two of water. Using a foil sling or silicone helper handles, lower the pan onto the trivet.

3. High pressure for 6 minutes. Close and lock the lid and select High Pressure for 6 minutes.

4. Pressure Release. Once the Cooking Time: is complete, quick release the pressure. Unlock and remove the lid.

5. Let cool for a few minutes before carefully lifting out the dish with oven mitts or tongs. Scoop out portions to serve.

Nutrition: Calories 275 Fat 19 g Carbohydrates 19 g Sugar 4 g Protein 14 g Cholesterol 60 mg

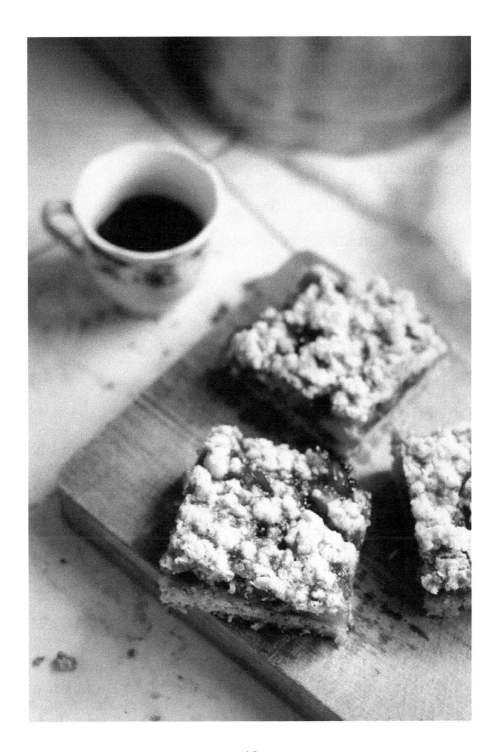

Almond-Date Energy Bites

Preparation Time: 5 minutes

Cooking Time: 15 minutes

Servings: 24

Ingredients:

- 1 cup dates, pitted
- 1 cup unsweetened shredded coconut
- ¼ cup chia seeds
- ¾ cup ground almonds
- ¼ cup cocoa nibs, or non-dairy chocolate chips

Directions:

1. Purée everything in a food processor until crumbly and sticking together, pushing down the sides whenever necessary to keep it blending. If you don't have a food processor, you can mash soft Medjool dates. But if you're using harder baking dates, you'll have to soak them and then try to purée them in a blender.

2. Form the mix into 24 balls and place them on a baking sheet lined with parchment or waxed paper.

Put in the fridge to set for about 15 minutes. Use the softest dates you can find. Medjool dates are the best for this purpose. The hard dates you see in the baking aisle of your supermarket are going to take a long time to blend up. If you use those, try soaking them in water for at least an hour before you start, and then draining.

Nutrition: Calories 171 Fat 4 g Carbohydrates 7 g Sugar 7 g Protein 22 g Cholesterol 65 mg

Pumpkin Pie Cups (Pressure cooker)

Preparation Time: 5 minutes

Cooking Time: 6 minutes

Servings: 4-6

Ingredients:

- 1 cup canned pumpkin purée
- 1 cup nondairy milk
- 6 tablespoons unrefined sugar or pure maple syrup (less if using sweetened milk), plus more for sprinkling
- ¼ cup spelt flour or whole-grain flour
- ½ teaspoon pumpkin pie spice
- Pinch salt

Directions:

1. Preparing the Ingredients. In a medium bowl, stir together the pumpkin, milk, sugar, flour, pumpkin pie spice, and salt. Pour the mixture into 4 heat-proof ramekins. Sprinkle a bit more sugar on the top of each, if you like. Put a trivet in the bottom of your electric pressure cooker's cooking pot and pour in a cup or two of water. Place the ramekins

onto the trivet, stacking them if needed (3 on the bottom, 1 on top).

2. High pressure for 6 minutes. Close and lock the lid and select High Pressure for 6 minutes.

3. Pressure Release. Once the Cooking Time: is complete, quick release the pressure. Unlock and remove the lid. Let cool for a few minutes before carefully lifting out the ramekins with oven mitts or tongs. Let cool for at least 10 minutes before serving.

Nutrition: Calories 152 Fat 4 g Carbohydrates 4 g Sugar 8 g Protein 18 g Cholesterol 51 mg

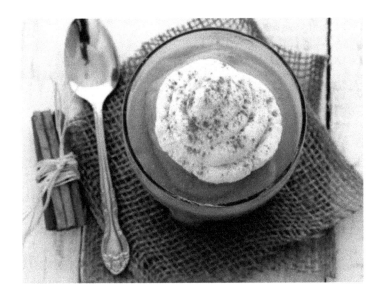

Fudgy Brownies (Pressure cooker)

Preparation Time: 10 minutes

Cooking Time: 5 minutes

Servings: 4-6

Ingredients:

- 3 ounces dairy-free dark chocolate
- 1 tablespoon coconut oil or vegan margarine
- ½ cup applesauce
- 2 tablespoons unrefined sugar
- 1/3 cup whole-grain flour
- ½ teaspoon baking powder
- Pinch salt

Directions:

1. Preparing the Ingredients. Put a trivet in your electric pressure cooker's cooking pot and pour in a cup or two of two of water. Select Sauté or Simmer. In a large heat-proof glass or ceramic bowl, combine the chocolate and coconut oil. Place the bowl over the top of your pressure cooker, as you would a double boiler. Stir occasionally until the chocolate is melted, then turn off the pressure

cooker. Stir the applesauce and sugar into the chocolate mixture. Add the flour, baking powder, and salt and stir just until combined. Pour the batter into 3 heat-proof ramekins. Put them in a heat-proof dish and cover with aluminum foil. Using a foil sling or silicone helper handles, lower the dish onto the trivet. (Alternately, cover each ramekin with foil and place them directly on the trivet, without the dish.)

2. High pressure for 6 minutes. Close and lock the lid, and select High Pressure for 5 minutes.

3. Pressure Release. Once the Cooking Time: is complete, quick release the pressure. Unlock and remove the lid.

4. Let cool for a few minutes before carefully lifting out the dish, or ramekins, with oven mitts or tongs. Let cool for a few minutes more before serving.

5. Top with fresh raspberries and an extra drizzle of melted chocolate.

Nutrition: Calories 256 Fat 29 g Carbohydrates 1 g Sugar 0.5 g Protein 11 g Cholesterol 84 mg

Chocolate Macaroons

Preparation Time: 10 minutes

Cooking Time: 15 minutes

Servings: 8

Ingredients:

- 1 cup unsweetened shredded coconut
- 2 tablespoons cocoa powder
- 2/3 cup coconut milk
- ¼ cup agave
- pinch of sea salt

Directions:

1. Preparing the Ingredients.
2. Preheat the oven to 350°F. Line a baking sheet with parchment paper. In a medium saucepan, cook all the ingredients over -medium-high heat until a firm dough is formed. Scoop the dough into balls and place on the baking sheet.
3. Bake for 15 minutes, remove from the oven, and let cool on the baking sheet.
4. Serve cooled macaroons or store in a tightly sealed container for up to

Nutrition: Calories 371 Fat 15 g Carbohydrates 7 g Sugar 2 g Protein 41 g Cholesterol 135 mg

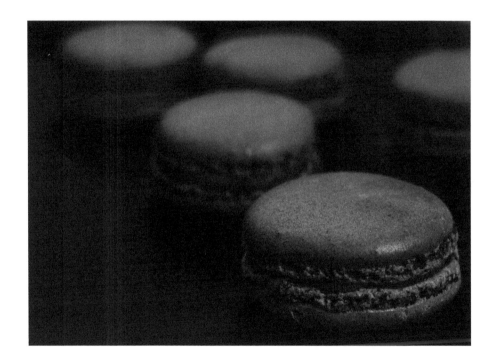

Express Coconut Flax Pudding

Preparation Time: 5 minutes

Cooking Time: 15 minutes

Servings: 4

Ingredients:

- 1 Tbsp. coconut oil softened
- 1 Tbsp. coconut cream
- 2 cups coconut milk canned
- 3/4 cup ground flax seed
- 4 Tbsp. coconut palm sugar (or to taste)

Directions:

1. Press SAUTÉ button on your Instant Pot
2. Add coconut oil, coconut cream, coconut milk, and ground flaxseed.
3. Stir about 5 - 10 minutes.
4. Lock lid into place and set on the MANUAL setting for 5 minutes.
5. When the timer beeps, press "Cancel" and carefully flip the Quick Release valve to let the pressure out.
6. Add the palm sugar and stir well.
7. Taste and adjust sugar to taste.

8. Allow pudding to cool down completely.

9. Place the pudding in an airtight container and refrigerate for up to 2 weeks.

Nutrition: Calories: 140 Fat: 2g Fiber: 23g Carbs: 22g Protein: 47g

Full-flavored Vanilla Ice Cream

Preparation Time: 5 minutes

Cooking Time: 20 minutes

Servings: 8

Ingredients:

- 1 1/2 cups canned coconut milk
- 1 cup coconut whipping cream
- 1 frozen banana cut into chunks
- 1 cup vanilla sugar
- 3 Tbsp. apple sauce
- 2 tsp pure vanilla extract
- 1 tsp Xanthan gum or agar-agar thickening agent

Directions:

1. Add all ingredients in a food processor; process until all ingredients combined well.
2. Place the ice cream mixture in a freezer-safe container with a lid over.
3. Freeze for at least 4 hours.
4. Remove frozen mixture to a bowl and beat with a mixer to break up the ice crystals.

5. Repeat this process 3 to 4 times.

6. Let the ice cream at room temperature for 15 minutes before serving.

Nutrition: Calories: 342 Fat: 15g Fiber: 11g Carbs: 8gProtein: 10g

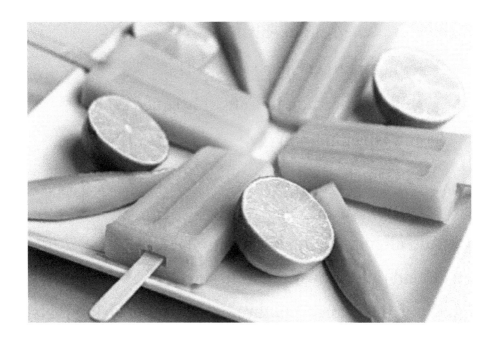

Seasoned Cinnamon Mango Popsicles

Preparation Time: 15 minutes

Cooking Time: 0 minute

Servings: 6

Ingredients:

- 1 1/2 cups of mango pulp
- 1 mango cut in cubes
- 1 cup brown sugar (packed)
- 2 Tbsp. lemon juice freshly squeezed
- 1 tsp cinnamon
- 1 pinch of salt

Directions:

1. Add all ingredients into your blender.
2. Blend until brown sugar dissolved.
3. Pour the mango mixture evenly in popsicle molds or cups.
4. Insert sticks into each mold.
5. Place molds in a freezer, and freeze for at least 5 to 6 hours.
6. Before serving, un-mold easy your popsicles placing molds under lukewarm water.

Nutrition: Calories: 423 Fat: 2g Fiber: 0g Carbs: 20g Protein: 33g

Strawberry Molasses Ice Cream

Preparation Time: 20 minutes

Cooking Time: 0 minute

Servings: 8

Ingredients:

- 1 lb. strawberries
- 3/4 cup coconut palm sugar (or granulated sugar)
- 1 cup coconut cream
- 1 Tbsp. molasses
- 1 tsp balsamic vinegar
- 1/2 tsp agar-agar
- 1/2 tsp pure strawberry extract

Directions:

1. Add strawberries, date sugar, and the balsamic vinegar in a blender; blend until completely combined.
2. Place the mixture in the refrigerator for one hour.
3. In a mixing bowl, beat the coconut cream with an electric mixer to make a thick mixture.

4. Add molasses, balsamic vinegar, agar-agar, and beat for further one minute or until combined well.

5. Keep frozen in a freezer-safe container (with plastic film and lid over).

Nutrition: Calories: 110 Fat: 31g Fiber: 18g Carbs: 15g Protein: 12g

Strawberry-Mint Sorbet

Preparation Time: 10 minutes

Cooking Time: 5 minutes

Servings: 6

Ingredients:

- 1 cup of granulated sugar
- 1 cup of orange juice
- 1 lb. frozen strawberries
- 1 tsp pure peppermint extract

Directions:

1. Add sugar and orange juice in a saucepan.
2. Stir over high heat and boil for 5 minutes or until sugar dissolves.
3. Remove from the heat and let it cool down.
4. Add strawberries into a blender, and blend until smooth.
5. Pour syrup into strawberries, add peppermint extract and stir until all ingredients combined well.
6. Transfer mixture to a storage container, cover tightly, and freeze until ready to serve.

Nutrition: Calories: 257 Fat: 13g Fiber: 37g Carbs: 11g Protein: 8g

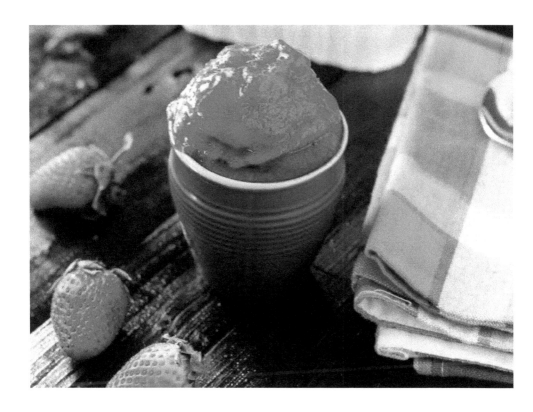

Keto Chocolate Brownies

Preparation Time: 15 minutes

Cooking Time: 15 minutes

Servings: 4

Ingredients:

- ¼ t. of the following:
- salt
- baking soda
- ½ c. of the following:
- sweetener of your choice
- coconut flour
- vegetable oil
- water
- ¼ c. of the following:
- cocoa powder
- almond milk yogurt
- 1 tbsp. ground flax
- 1 t. vanilla extract

Directions:

1. Bring the oven to 350 heat setting.

2. Mix the ground flax, vanilla, yogurt, oil, and water; set to the side for 10 minutes.

3. Line an oven-safe 8x8 baking dish with parchment paper.

4. After 10 minutes have passed, add coconut flour, cocoa powder, sweetener, baking soda, and salt.

5. Bake for 15 minutes; make sure that you placed it in the center. When they come out, they will look underdone.

6. Place in the refrigerator and let them firm up overnight.

Nutrition: Calories: 208 Fat: 3g Fiber: 4g Carbs: 7g Protein: 27g

Chocolate Fat Bomb

Preparation Time: 5 minutes

Cooking Time: 0 minutes

Servings: 14

Ingredients:

- 1 tbsp. liquid sweetener of your choice.
- ¼ c. of the following:
- coconut oil, melted
- cocoa powder
- ½ c. almond butter

Directions:

1. Mix the ingredients in a medium bowl until smooth. Pour into the candy molds or ice cube trays.
2. Put in the freezer to set.
3. Store in freezer.

Nutrition: Calories: 241 Fat: 2g Fiber: 16g Carbs: 9g Protein: 22g

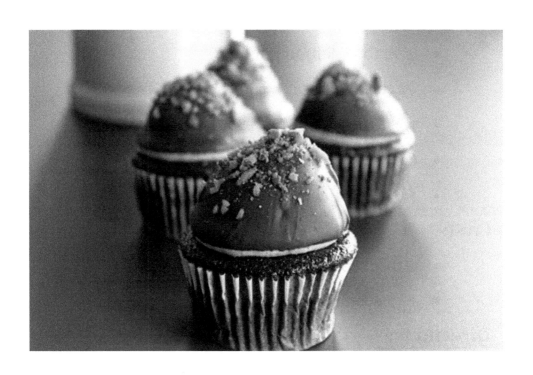

Vanilla Cheesecake

Preparation Time: 3 hours 20 minutes

Cooking Time: 0 minute

Servings: 10

Ingredients:

- 1 tbsp. vanilla extract,
- 2 ½ tbsp. lemon juice
- ½ c. coconut oil
- 1/8 t. stevia powder
- 6 tbsp. coconut milk
- 1 ½ c. blanched almonds soaked

Crust:

- 2 tbsp. coconut oil
- 1 ½ c. almonds

Directions:

For the Crust:

1. In a food processor, add the almonds and coconut oil and pulse until crumbles start to form.
2. Line a 7-inch spring form pan with parchment paper and firmly press the crust into the bottom.
3. For the Sauce:

4. Bring a saucepan of water to a boil and soak the almonds for 2 hours. Drain and shake to dry.

5. Next, add the almonds to the food processor and blend until completely smooth.

6. Add vanilla, lemon, coconut oil, stevia, and coconut milk and blend until smooth.

7. Pour over the crust and freeze overnight or for a minimum of 3 hours.

8. Serve and enjoy.

Nutrition: Calories: 267 Fat: 13g Fiber: 14g Carbs: 17g Protein: 10g

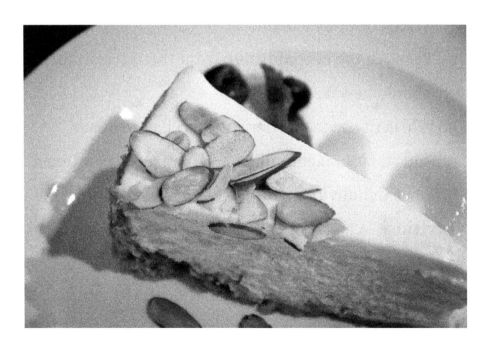

Chocolate Mousse

Preparation Time: 5 minutes

Cooking Time: 0 minute

Servings: 2

Ingredients:

- 6 drops liquid stevia extract
- ½ t. cinnamon
- 3 tbsp. cocoa powder, unsweetened
- 1 c. coconut milk

Directions:

1. On the day before, place the coconut milk into the refrigerator overnight.
2. Remove the coconut milk from the refrigerator; it should be very thick.
3. Whisk in cocoa powder with an electric mixer.
4. Add stevia and cinnamon and whip until combined.
5. Place in individual bowls and serve and enjoy.

Nutrition: Calories: 130 Fat: 5g Fiber: 3g Carbs: 6gProtein: 7g

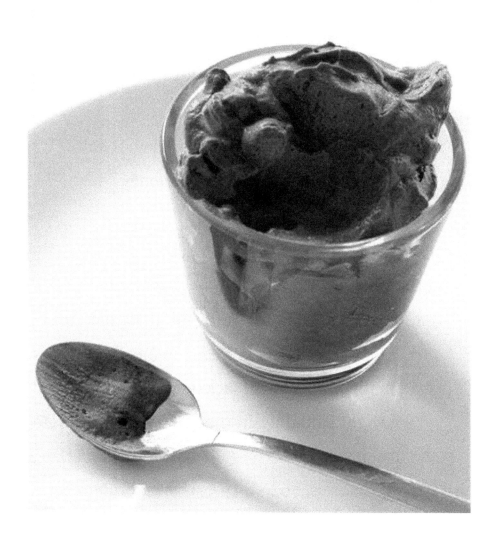

Tahini Miso Dressing

Preparation Time: 10 minutes

Cooking Time: 0 minute

Servings: 2

Ingredients:

- ¼ cup tahini
- 1 tablespoon tamari or low-sodium soy sauce
- 1 tablespoon white miso
- 1 tablespoon freshly squeezed lemon juice
- 1 tablespoon maple syrup or honey
- ¼ cup warm water
- Freshly ground black pepper

Directions:

1. In a small bowl, whisk the tahini, tamari, miso, lemon juice, and maple syrup together. Whisk in the water and black pepper. Store in an airtight container in the refrigerator for up to six months.

Nutrition: Calories: 76 Fat: 6g Carbs: 5g Protein: 2g

Balsamic Roasted Tomatoes

Preparation Time: 10 minutes

Cooking Time: 4 hours

Servings: 6

Ingredients:

- 6 medium tomatoes or 1 pint cherry tomatoes
- ¼ cup, plus 1 tablespoon olive oil
- Kosher salt
- Freshly ground black pepper
- 2 teaspoons balsamic vinegar

Directions:

1. Preheat the oven to 300°F. Put your rimmed baking sheet with parchment paper.

2. Wash and dry the tomatoes and halve them crosswise. Put them cut side up on the parchment paper, and drizzle them with ¼ cup of olive oil, allowing the oil to pool on the parchment paper. Sprinkle with the salt and pepper.

3. Roast for 3 to 4 hours, or until the edges of the tomatoes are puckered and the cut surface is a little dry.

4. Sprinkle with the balsamic vinegar and let cool on the baking sheet.

5. Pack into an airtight container, and pour any excess oil from the parchment paper on top. Add the remaining 1 tablespoon of oil to the container. Seal and refrigerate for up to one month.

Nutrition: Calories: 123 Fat: 12g Carbs: 5g Protein: 1g

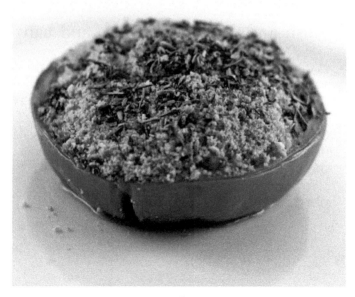

Lentil Potato Salad

Preparation Time: 10 minutes

Cooking Time: 25 minutes

Servings: 2

Ingredients:

- ½ cup beluga lentils
- 8 fingerling potatoes
- 1 cup thinly sliced scallions
- ¼ cup halved cherry tomatoes
- ¼ cup Lemon Vinaigrette
- Kosher salt, to taste
- Freshly ground black pepper, to taste

Directions:

1. Pour 2 cups of water to simmer in a small pot and add the lentils. Cover and simmer for 20 to 25 minutes, or until the lentils are tender. Drain and set aside to cool.

2. While the lentils are cooking, bring a medium pot of well-salted water to a boil and add the potatoes. Low heat to simmer and cook for about 15 minutes, or until the potatoes are

tender. Drain. Once cool enough to handle, slice or halve the potatoes.

3. Place the lentils on a serving plate and top with the potatoes, scallions, and tomatoes. Drizzle with the vinaigrette and season with the salt and pepper.

Nutrition: Calories: 400 Fat: 26g Carbs: 39g Protein: 7g

Bok Choy–Asparagus Salad

Preparation Time: 20 minutes

Cooking Time: 0 minute

Servings: 4

Ingredients:

- 4 cups coarsely chopped baby bok Choy
- 1½ cups asparagus, trimmed and cut into 1½-inch lengths
- 1 cup cauliflower rice
- 1 cup strawberries, chopped into bite-size chunks
- 1 mango, peeled and diced
- ½ cup scallions, sliced into 1-inch lengths
- ¼ cup Lemon Vinaigrette

Directions:

1. In a large bowl, combine the bok choy, asparagus, cauliflower rice, strawberries, mango, and scallions. Drizzle with the vinaigrette and gently toss.

Nutrition: Calories: 210 Fat: 14g Carbs: 21g Protein: 3g

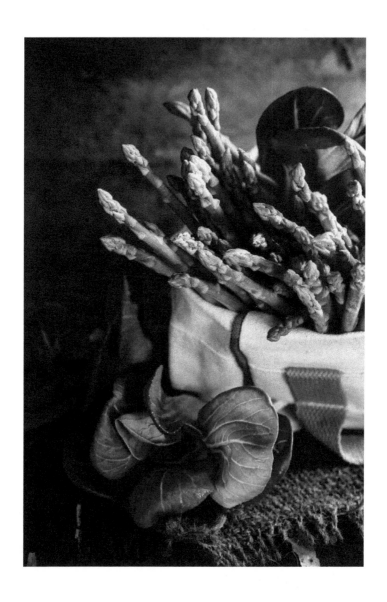

Lemony Romaine and Avocado Salad

Preparation Time: 15 minutes

Cooking Time: 0 minute

Servings: 6

Ingredients:

- 1 head romaine lettuce
- ½ cup pomegranate seeds
- ¼ cup pine nuts
- ¼ cup Lemon Vinaigrette
- 2 avocados
- Freshly ground black pepper

Directions:

2. Wash your vegetables and spin-dry then slice the leaves into bite-size pieces. Transfer the leaves in a large bowl, and toss with the pomegranate seeds, pine nuts, and half of the vinaigrette.

3. Slice the avocados in half. Remove the pit from each and slice the avocados into long thin

slices. Using a large spoon, carefully scoop the slices out of the peel.

4. Arrange your avocado slices on top of the lettuce in the bowl, and drizzle half of the remaining dressing over them. Carefully toss using your hands or a large metal spoon. Add the remaining dressing as needed.

5. Finish with a few sprinkles of pepper.

Nutrition: Calories: 217 Fat: 20g Carbs: 11g Protein 3g

Aloha Mango-Pineapple Smoothie

Preparation Time: 10 minutes

Cooking Time: 0 minute

Servings: 2

Ingredients:

- 1 large navel orange, peeled and quartered
- 1 cup frozen pineapple chunks
- 1 cup frozen mango chunks
- 1 tablespoon freshly squeezed lime juice
- ½ cup plain Greek yogurt
- ½ cup milk or coconut milk
- 1 tablespoon chia seeds (optional)
- 3 or 4 ice cubes

Directions:

1. Transfer all your ingredients in a blender and blend until smooth. If necessary, add additional milk or water to thin the smoothie to your preferred consistency.

Nutrition: Calories: 158 Fat: 1g Carbs: 35g Protein: 7g

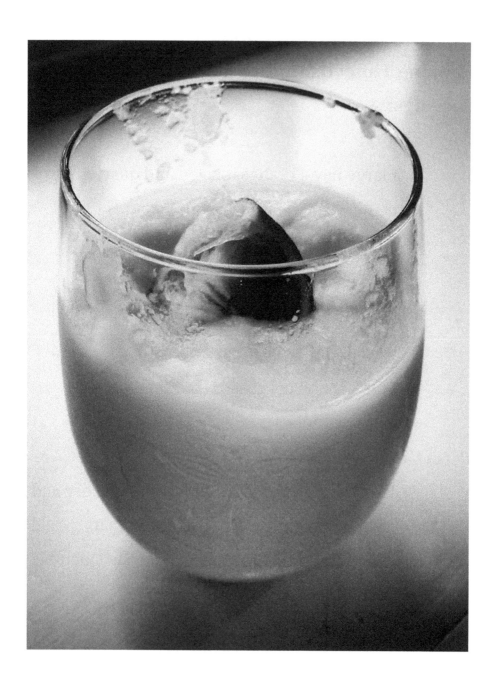

Delicious Lentil Soup

Preparation Time: 15 Minutes

Cooking Time: 25 Minutes

Servings: 4

Ingredients:

- 1 tbsp. Olive Oil
- 4 cups Vegetable Stock
- 1 Onion, finely chopped
- 2 Carrots, medium
- 1 cup Lentils, dried
- 1 tsp. Cumin

Directions:

1. To make this healthy soup, first, you need to heat the oil in a medium-sized skillet over medium heat.
2. Once the oil becomes hot, stir in the cumin and then the onions.
3. Sauté those for 3 minutes or until the onion is slightly transparent and cooked.
4. To this, add the carrots and toss them well.
5. Next, stir in the lentils. Mix well.

6. Now, pour in the vegetable stock and give a good stir until everything comes together.

7. As the soup mixture starts to boil, reduce the heat and allow it to simmer for 10 minutes while keeping the pan covered.

8. Turn off the heat and then transfer the mixture to a bowl.

9. Finally, blend it with an immersion blender or in a high-speed blender for 1 minute or until you get a rich, smooth mixture.

10. Serve it hot and enjoy.

Nutrition: Calories: 251 Kcal Protein: 14g Carbohydrates: 41.3g Fat: 4.1g

Trail Mix

Preparation Time: 10 Minutes

Cooking Time: 10 Minutes

Servings: 2

Ingredients:

- 1 cup Walnuts, raw
- 2 cups Tart Cherries, dried
- 1 cup Pumpkin Seeds, raw
- 1 cup Almonds, raw
- ½ cup Vegan Dark Chocolate
- 1 cup Cashew

Directions:

1. First, mix all the ingredients needed to make the trail mix in a large mixing bowl until combined well.
2. Store in an air-tight container.

Nutrition: Calories: 596 Kcal Protein: 17.5g Carbohydrates: 46.1g Fat: 39.5g

Flax Crackers

Preparation Time: 5 Minutes

Cooking Time: 60 Minutes

Servings: 4 to 6

Ingredients:

- 1 cup Flaxseeds, whole
- 2 cups Water
- ¾ cup Flaxseeds, grounded
- 1 tsp. Sea Salt
- ½ cup Chia Seeds
- 1 tsp. Black Pepper
- ½ cup Sunflower Seeds

Directions:

1. Using a large bowl, you need to put all your ingredients then mix them well. Soak them in a water for about 10 to 15 minutes.

2. After that, transfer the mixture to a parchment paper-lined baking sheet and spread it evenly. Tip: Make sure the paper lines the edges as well.

3. Next, bake it for 60 minutes at 350 °F.

4. Once the time is up, flip the entire bar and take off the parchment paper.

5. Bake for half an hour or until it becomes crispy and browned.

6. Allow it to cool completely and then break it down.

Nutrition: Calories: 251cal Proteins: 9.2g Carbohydrates: 14.9g Fat: 16g

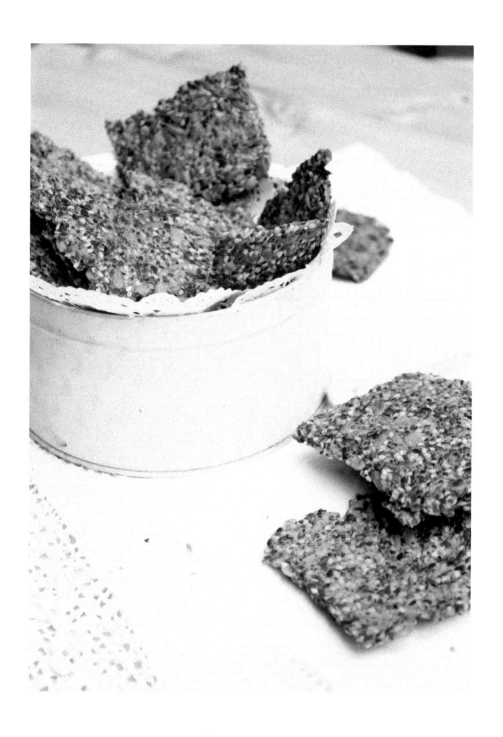

Crunchy Granola

Preparation Time: 10 Minutes

Cooking Time: 20 Minutes

Servings: 1

Ingredients:

- ½ cup Oats
- Dash of Salt
- 2 tbsp. Vegetable Oil
- 3 tbsp. Maple Syrup
- 1/3 cup Apple Cider Vinegar
- ½ cup Almonds
- 1 tsp. Cardamom, grounded

Directions:

1. Preheat the oven to 375 °F.
2. After that, mix oats, pistachios, salt, and cardamom in a large bowl.
3. Next, spoon in the vegetable oil and maple syrup to the mixture.
4. Then, transfer the mixture to a parchment-paper-lined baking sheet.

5. Bake them for 13 minutes or until the mixture is toasted. Tip: Check on them now and then. Spread it out well.

6. Return the sheet to the oven for further ten minutes.

7. From your oven remove the sheet and allow it to cool completely.

8. Serve and enjoy.

Nutrition: Calories: 763Kcal Proteins: 12.9g Carbohydrates: 64.8g Fat: 52.4g

Chickpea Scramble Bowl

Preparation Time: 10 Minutes

Cooking Time: 10 Minutes

Servings: Makes 2 Bowl

Ingredients:

- ¼ of 1 Onion, diced
- 15 oz. Chickpeas
- 2 Garlic cloves, minced
- ½ tsp. Turmeric
- ½ tsp. Black Pepper
- ½ tsp. Extra Virgin Olive Oil
- ½ tsp. Salt

Directions:

1. Begin by placing the chickpeas in a large bowl along with a bit of water.
2. Soak for few minutes and then mash the chickpeas lightly with a fork while leaving some of them in the whole form.
3. Next, spoon in the turmeric, pepper, and salt to the bowl. Mix well.

4. Then, heat oil in a medium-sized skillet over medium-high heat.

5. Once the oil becomes hot, stir in the onions.

6. Sauté the onions for 3 to 4 minutes or until softened.

7. Then, add the garlic and cook for further 1 minute or until aromatic.

8. After that, stir in the mashed chickpeas. Cook for another 4 minutes or until thickened.

9. Serve along with micro greens. Place the greens at the bottom, followed by the scramble, and top it with cilantro or parsley.

Nutrition: Calories: 801Kcal Proteins: 41.5g Carbohydrates: 131.6g Fat: 14.7g

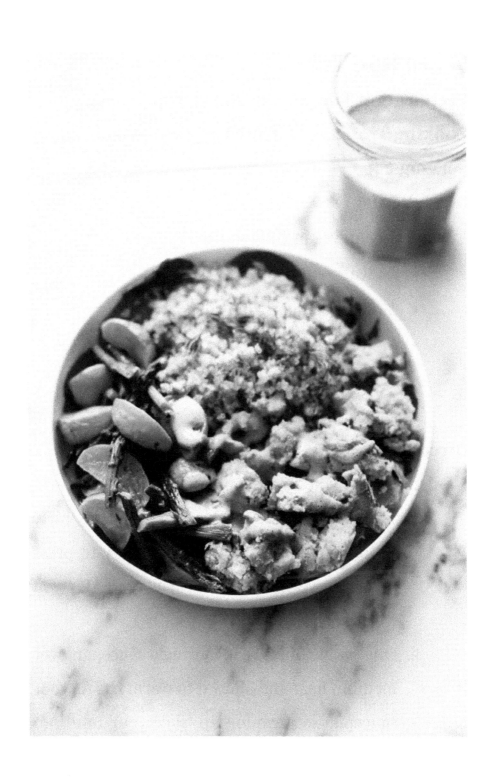

Vegan BBQ Tofu

Preparation Time: 10 minutes

Cooking Time: 40 minutes

Servings: 3

Ingredients:

- ¼ cup vegan BBQ sauce
- ¼ teaspoon pepper
- ¼ teaspoon garlic powder
- ¼ teaspoon salt
- 1 tablespoon grape seed oil
- 1 pack firm tofu

Directions:

1. Before you begin cooking your tofu, you will want to press it. Generally, this will take thirty to forty-five minutes. If possible, try to press the tofu overnight so that it is ready for you when you need it.

2. Once your tofu is ready, bring a saucepan over medium heat and allow it to warm up. As your saucepan is warming up, slice your tofu into small pieces. Put a 1 tablespoon of oil and

spread your tofu across the pan. At this point, season your tofu and cook for five minutes. Be sure to flip each piece of tofu until it is a nice golden-brown colour all over.

3. Finally, remove the tofu from the pan and cover it in BBQ sauce. This meal is excellent alone or with your favourite grain or vegetable.

Nutrition: Calories: 290, Fat: 64 g, Carbs: 25 g, Protein: 20 g

Broccoli over Orzo

Preparation Time: 10 minutes

Cooking Time: 25 minutes

Servings: 3

Ingredients:

- 3 teaspoons olive oil
- 4 garlic cloves, smashed
- 2 cups broccoli florets
- 4½ ounces orzo pasta
- ¼ teaspoon salt
- ¼ teaspoon pepper

Directions:

1. Start off by preparing your broccoli. You can do this by trimming the stems off and slicing the broccoli into small, bite-size pieces. If you want, go ahead and season with salt.

2. Next, you will want to steam your broccoli over a little bit of water until it is cooked through. Once the broccoli is cooked, chop it up into even smaller pieces.

3. When the broccoli is done, cook your pasta according to the directions provided on the box. Once this is done, drain the water and then place the pasta back into the pot.

4. With the pasta and broccoli done, place it back into the pot with the garlic. Stir everything together well and cook until the garlic turns a nice golden colour. Be sure to stir everything to combine your meal well. Serve warm and enjoy a simple dinner!

Nutrition: Calories: 310 Fat: 4 g Carbs: 35 g Protein: 10 g

Mango Pineapple Hoisin Sauce

Preparation Time: 10 minutes

Cooking Time: 10 minutes

Servings: 2

Ingredients:

- 1 ½ cups fresh mango juice or pureed mango
- ⅔ cup vegan hoisin sauce
- 4 tablespoons brown rice vinegar
- 1 cup fresh pineapple juice
- ½ cup tamari or soy sauce
- 2 tablespoons Sriracha sauce

Directions:

1. Use a pan and heat oil over medium heat.
2. Add all the ingredients and stir constantly.
3. Simmer until the mixture thickens.

Nutrition: Calories: 125 Fat: 2 g Carbs: 8 g Protein: 4.3 g

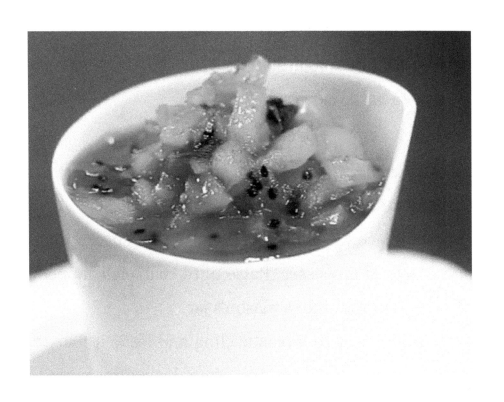

Sriracha Sauce

Preparation Time: 20 minutes

Cooking Time: 10 minutes

Servings: 2

Ingredients

- 15 red Fresno chilies, chopped into chunks
- ½ tablespoon salt
- 4 garlic cloves
- ¼ cup apple cider or white vinegar
- 2 tablespoons raw sugar

Directions:

1. Place the chilies, garlic, salt and sugar into a food processor. Pulse until coarsely chopped. Transfer into a mason's jar.

2. Cover with a plastic cling and leave it for 5-7 days to ferment. Stir often during this period. In 3-4 days, you will see some bubbles appearing.

3. Transfer the contents of the jar into a blender. Add vinegar and blend until smooth.

4. Transfer into a saucepan after passing through a wire mesh strainer.

5. Bring to a boil on high heat.

6. When it starts boiling, reduce the heat and simmer for 5 minutes. Remove from heat and cool.

7. Transfer into a flip top bottle. Refrigerate until use.

Nutrition: Calories: 90 Fat: 6 g Carbs: 5 g Protein: 1 g

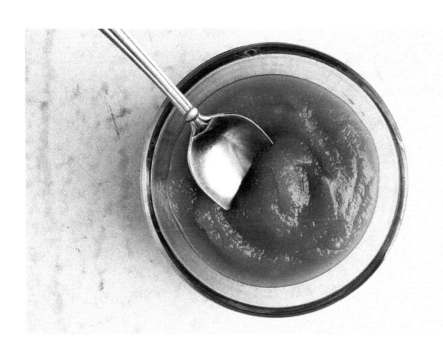

White Sauce (Béchamel)

Preparation Time: 10 minutes

Cooking Time: 12 minutes

Servings: 2

Ingredients:

- 6 tablespoons olive oil
- 4 cups soymilk or any other non-dairy milk of your choice
- 5 tablespoons all-purpose flour
- Sea salt to taste
- Black pepper to taste

Directions:

1. Place a heavy pot over a medium heat. Add oil. When the oil is heated, add sifted flour into the pan. Stir constantly for about a minute. It will begin to change colour; be careful not to burn it!

2. Pour in the milk, stirring constantly. Keep stirring until thick.

3. Simmer until the thickness you desire is nearly achieved. This is because the sauce thickens further as it cools.

4. Turn off the heat. Add salt, pepper and any other herbs and spices if you desire.

Lightning Source UK Ltd.
Milton Keynes UK
UKHW020105241222
414375UK00001B/16